How to
Boost Your
Metabolism

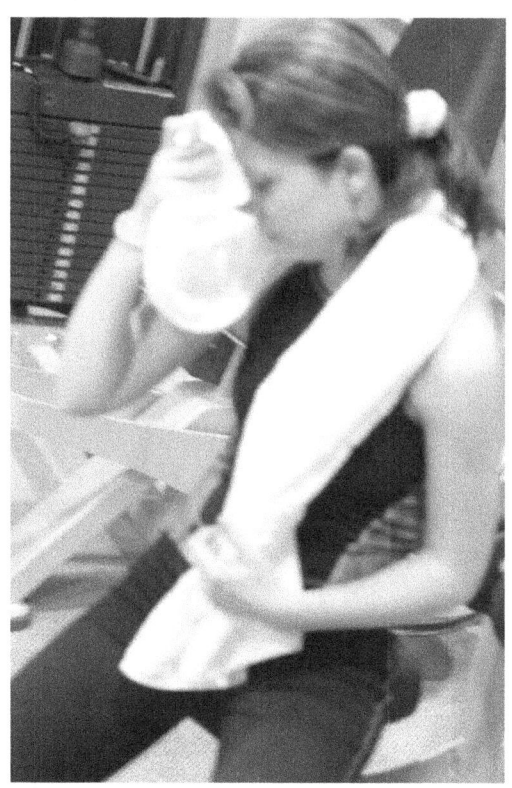

By
James B. Driscoll

Table of Contents

Introduction

Metabolism. There isn't perhaps a more frequently used word in the weight loss (and weight gain) vocabulary than this.

Indeed, it's not uncommon to overhear people talking about their struggles – or triumphs – over the holiday bulge or *love handles* in terms of whether their metabolism is working, or not.

Doctors, too, often refer to metabolism when they try and explain why starvation and water-loss diets aren't scientifically of medically responsible; since, alas, they do not influence or take into account metabolism (there's that word again!).

So, for all of the usage that this rather daunting and biologically-charged word enjoys in our world, you'd comfortably assume that people understand it, right?

Or, at least, they have some fundamental information when it comes to how to speed *up* their metabolism, right?

Wrong!

Towards Understanding Metabolism

Regrettably, many people simply *don't* understand the concept of metabolism and metabolic change. This, equally as regrettably, is hardly their fault.

There is so much information floating around out there, much of it over the 'net or through a "friend of a friend who has a personal trainer", that there's bound to be some confusion and conflicting messages.

Furthermore, many people (quite understandably) mistake their own weight gain and loss episodes as a matter of metabolic change. Sometimes this is true, and sometimes it isn't.

For example, as we will discuss in this book, there are scientific ways to increase the rate of metabolic change, and thus enable the body to burn more calories.

Eating *certain foods* more frequently is one way to do this (again, we look closer at these in this book). Yet another way to visibly lose weight – at least on a perceived, temporary level – is to sit in a steam room for a few hours.

Whereas the former method (eating the right foods) is a real, *proven* weight loss method through increased metabolic change, the latter method (the steam room) is just temporary because the lost weight is merely water, and will return as swiftly as it "melted away".

The point to remember here is that some people mistake their own weight loss attempts as being related to metabolic change; and, as you can see with the steam room example, that isn't always the case.

Low Fat Labels

Another big reason that people don't have clear, consistent information on this topic is because, unfortunately, there are a lot of food and supplement companies on the market who don't *want* you to know fact from fiction.

They want you to believe that constantly buying "low fat" foods is going to somehow speed up your metabolism.

While, yes, *some* low fat foods can play a role in an overall eating program that is designed to speed up metabolism, merely eating foods that come from packaging that screams "LOW FAT!" won't do anything.

In fact, believe it or not, but many people actually *gain* weight when they eat too many "low fat" products. Many of these products are laden with calories from carbohydrates or proteins (which are *still* calories and *still* must be burned off or they turn into body fat).

As you can see, and probably *feel* from years of trying to unravel this whole metabolic mystery, this is a confusing, stressful, and indeed, potentially depressing situation.

Each year, tens of millions of people attempt to retake control over their health and the shape of their body; and each year, tens of millions of people feel that they've "failed" because, try as they might, they just can't speed up their metabolism.

This book is the antidote to that way of thinking and feeling because the perceived failure is *not* a failure in any of these hard working dieters and exercisers (of which you may be one).

The failure is with the medical and nutritional sector as a whole, which has simply not provided people with the information that they *need to know* in order to speed up their metabolism.

And given the size of the nutritional field and the fact that so much of it is influenced by money-making enterprises (not all of the field, of course, but enough of it to make a difference), there's really no sense in playing a "wait and see" game for when clear, consistent, and helpful information starts to flow out to people like us.

What's Inside...

And that's why this book exists. It's been created for the millions of everyday people like us who simply want to know how to speed up metabolism, and how to lose weight the right, healthy, and responsible way. We want to know:

- **What the heck a metabolism is, and what role it really plays on weight loss and gain**

- **The proven, scientific ways to speed up metabolism - not myths and fitness club "speculation"; but the *real deal*.**

- **Specific diet and food items and promote a faster metabolism, so that once unwanted weight has been lost, it can be *kept off* through a responsible eating plan.**

And in the pages ahead, that's precisely what we cover!

Part 1: What is Metabolism?

Some people think that the metabolism is a kind of organ, or a body part, that influences digestion.

Actually, the metabolism isn't any particular body part.

It's the *process* by which the body converts food into energy.

Hence, you've likely heard of the phrase *metabolic process* used synonymously with the term *metabolism*, because they both mean the same thing.

The Medical Mumbo Jumbo

This isn't a complicated medical text (which should be great news to most of you!), and so we don't need to spend an unnecessary amount of time and space focusing on the layered complexity of the human body and its extraordinary intelligence.

Yet without drilling deeply into medical details -- which are not relevant for our general understanding purposes -- it's helpful to briefly look at the biological mechanisms behind metabolism.

Metabolism, as mentioned above, is the process of transforming food (e.g. nutrients) into fuel (e.g. energy). The body uses this energy to conduct a vast array of essential functions.

In fact, your ability to read this page – literally – is driven by your metabolism.

If you had *no* metabolism – that is, if you had no metabolic process that was converting food into energy – then you wouldn't be able to move.

In fact, long before you realized that you couldn't move a finger or lift your foot, your internal processes would have stopped; because the basic building blocks of life – circulating blood, transforming oxygen into carbon dioxide, expelling potentially lethal wastes through the kidneys and so on – *all of these* depend on metabolism.

Keep this in mind the next time you hear someone say that they have a *slow metabolism*.

While they may struggle with unwanted weight gain due to metabolic factors, they certainly have a *functioning metabolism*.

If they didn't, they wouldn't even be able to speak (because that, too, requires energy that comes from, you guessed it: metabolism!).

It's also interesting to note that, while we conveniently refer to the *metabolic process* as if it were a single function, it's really a catch-all term for countless functions that are taking place inside the body. Every second of every minute of every day of your life – even, of course, when you sleep – numerous chemical conversions are taking place through metabolism, or metabolic functioning.

In a certain light, the metabolism has been referred to as a harmonizing process that manages to achieve two critical bodily functions that, in a sense, seem to be at odds with each other.

The first function is creating tissue and cells. Each moment, our bodies are creating more cells to replace dead or dysfunctional cells.

For example, if you cut your finger, your body (if it's functioning properly) will begin – without even wasting a moment or asking your permission –the process of creating skin cells to clot the blood and start the healing process. This creation process is indeed a metabolic response, and is called *anabolism*.

On the other hand, there is the exact *opposite* activity taking place in other parts of the body. Instead of building cells and tissue through metabolism, the body is breaking down energy so that the body can do what it's supposed to do.

For example, as you aerobically exercise, your body temperature rises as your heart beat increases and remains with a certain range.

As this happens, your body requires more oxygen; and as such, your breathing increases as you intake more H^2O. All of this, as you can imagine, requires additional energy.

After all, if your body couldn't adjust to this enhanced requirement for oxygen (both taking it in and getting rid of it in the form of carbon dioxide), you would collapse!

Presuming, of course, that you *aren't* overdoing it, your body will instead begin converting food (e.g. calories) into energy. And this process, as you know, is a metabolic process, and is called *catabolism*.

So as you can see, the metabolism is a *constant* process that takes care of two seemingly opposite function: anabolism that uses energy to *create* cells, and catabolism that *breaks down* cells to create energy.

Indeed, it's in this way that the metabolism earns its reputation as a harmonizer. It brings together these apparently conflicting functions, and does so in an optimal way that enables the body to create cells as needed, and break them down, again as needed.

Metabolism and Weight Loss

By now, you already have a sense of how metabolism relates to weight loss (catabolic metabolism, or breaking cells down and transforming them into energy).

To understand this process even more clearly, we can introduce a very important player in the weight loss game: the *calorie*.

Calories

Calories are simply units of measure. They aren't actually *things* in and of themselves; they are labels for other things, just like how an inch really isn't anything, but it measures the distance between two points.

So what do calories measure?

Easy: they measure *energy*.

Yup, the evil calorie – the bane of the dieter's existence – is really just a 3-syllable label for energy.

And it's important to highlight this, because the body itself, despite its vast intelligence (much of which medical science cannot yet understand, only appreciate in awe) does not really do a very intelligent job of distinguishing good energy from bad.

Actually, to be blunt, the body doesn't *care* about where the energy comes from. Let's explore this a little more, because it's very important to the overall understanding of how to boost your metabolism, particularly when we look at food choices.

In our choice-laden grocery stores, with dozens of varieties of foods – hundreds, perhaps – there seems to be a fairly clear awareness of what's *good* food, and what's *bad* or *junk* food.

For example, we don't need a book to remind us that, all else being equal, a plum is a *good* food, whereas a tub of thick and creamy double-fudge ice cream is a *bad* food.

Not bad tasting, of course; but, really, you won't find many fit people eating a vat of ice cream a day, for obvious reasons. So what does this have to do with calories and energy?

It's this: while *you and I* can evaluate our food choices and say that something (like a plum) is a healthy source of energy, and something else (like a tub of ice cream) is an unhealthy source of energy, <u>*the body doesn't evaluate*</u>. Really.

It sounds strange and amazing, but the body really doesn't care. To the body, *energy is energy*. It takes whatever it gets, and doesn't really *know* that some foods are healthier than others. It's kind of like a garbage disposal: it takes what you put down it, whether it *should* go down or not.

So let's apply this to the body, and to weight gain. When the body receives a calorie – which, as we know, is merely a label for *energy* – it must do something with that energy.

In other words, putting all other nutrients and minerals aside, if a plum delivers 100 calories to the body, it *has* to accept those 100 calories. The same goes for 500 calories from a (small) tub of ice cream: those 500 calories *have* to be dealt with.

Now, the body does two things to that energy: it either metabolizes it via anabolism, or it metabolizes it via catabolism. That is, it will either convert the energy (calories) into cells/tissue, or it will use that energy (calories) to break down cells.

Now the link between calories/energy, metabolism, and weight loss becomes rather clear and direct.

When there is an excess of energy, and the body can't use this energy to deal with any needs at the time, **it will be forced to create cells with that extra energy.** It has to.

It doesn't necessarily *want* to, but after figuring out that the energy can't be used to do anything (such as help you exercise or digest some food), it *has* to turn it into cells through anabolism.

And those extra cells? Yup, you guessed it: added weight!

In a nutshell (and nuts have lots of calories by the way, so watch out and eat them in small portions...), the whole calorie/metabolism/weight gain thing is really just about excess energy. When there are too many calories in the body – that is, when there's *too much energy* from food – then the body transforms those calories into *stuff*.

And that *stuff*, most of the time, is fat. Sometimes, of course, those extra calories are transformed into muscle; and this is usually a good thing for those watching their weight or trying to maintain an optimal body fat ratio.

In fact, because muscles require calories to maintain, people with strong muscle tone *burn calories* without actually doing anything; their metabolism burns it for them.

This is the primary reason why exercising and building lean muscle is part of an overall program to boost your metabolism; because the more lean muscle you have, the more *places* excess calories can go *before* they're turned into fat.

A Final Word About Fat

There's a nasty rumor floating around out there that fat cells are *permanent*. And the nastiest thing about this rumor is that it's true.

Yes, most experts conceded that fat cells – once created – are there for life. Yet this doesn't spell doom and gloom to those of us who could stand to *drop a few pounds*. Because even though experts believe that fat cells are permanent, they also agree that fat cells can be *shrunk*. So even if the absolute number of fat cells in your body remains the same, their size – and hence their appearance and percentage of your overall weight – can be reduced.

Recap

So while we haven't gone into any medical detail – because we don't need to or want to – we have covered some key basics about metabolism. In fact, you probably know as much about metabolism now as many so-called experts.

The bottom line is simply that metabolism represents a process – countless processes, in fact – that convert food into energy. When this process creates cells, it's called anabolism. When this process breaks cells down, it's called catabolism.

For people trying to lose weight, it's important to experience *catabolism*. That is, it's important convert food into energy that is used to break cells down.

Catabolism is also important because it prevents excess energy (calories) from being stored by the body.

Remember: when the body has too many calories – regardless of what food source those calories came from – it can only do two things. It can desperately try and see if you have any energy needs (like maybe you're running a marathon at the time).

Or, more often, it will *have* to store those calories. It has no choice. And unless you have lean muscle that is gobbling up those excess calories, you'll be adding fat.

The remainder of this book, however, is going to point you in the *opposite* direction. You'll learn various techniques, tips, and strategies to boost your metabolism.

And then, in the latter part of this book, you'll be introduced to some metabolism-boosting foods that you'll surely want to add to your regular eating regimen.

Part 2: Tips, Techniques, and Strategies for Boosting Your Metabolism

If you're reading this book, chances are that you've tried – at least *once* in your life – to boost your metabolism.

Perhaps (like most of us) you weren't quite certain what a metabolism *was*, and perhaps (again, like most of us) you probably didn't quite know all that you needed to know in order to accomplish your goals.

Maybe you started a rigorous exercise program of jogging and muscle toning.

Or maybe you started eating several small portions a day, rather than three large traditional *meal-sized* portions.

Or maybe you started taking all kinds of supplements that promised to boost your metabolism.

The thing is, is that *all* of these methods can indeed work.

Really: exercise, eating strategically, and ensuring that your body has catabolism-friendly supplements are but three of many generally good ideas.

So what's the problem?

The problem is that many of us have no real scientific understanding of *what, how, or why* these methods boost metabolism.

Some of us, in fact, don't really even know if they work; we just think that they do.

For example, a person may start a vigorous exercise program that includes significant aerobic cardiovascular movement, such as jogging or cycling.

And indeed, after a week, that person may notice a drop in weight.

Yet is this due to a boosted metabolism? Maybe; maybe not. Could it be due to water loss through perspiration that hasn't been adequately replenished? Maybe or maybe not.

The point here is that many people – at risk to their health and wellness – don't quite understand the tips, strategies, and techniques of boosting their metabolism. And that's what we're going to rectify in this chapter.

In this book, you won't come across any casual information that *a friend of a friend heard on TV.* Nor will you be subjected to off-the-cuff information of how to boost your metabolism.

Rather, we're going to look at the popular, easy, fun (yes, believe it or not), and *successful* ways to boost your metabolism.

The popular and widely respected Internet publication *i-Village*[i] highlights 11 key ways to speed up metabolism. To most easily introduce and discuss them here, we've taken these 11 key ideas and broken them down into 3 broad categories:

1. **Exercise**
2. **Lifestyle**
3. **Diet**

As you go through each of the 11 key points, you'll certainly note that there is some overlap between them. For example, it's hard to imagine that introducing exercise into your life isn't, in many ways, a *lifestyle* choice.

Similarly, integrating all kinds of metabolism-boosting foods into your diet is surely going to influence how you spend your time (probably less time in fast food line-ups, for one!).

So with this being said, *please* don't get bogged down in the categories; they are merely provided here to help organize these points, and to help you easily refer to them in the future. The important thing for you to do is understand each of the 14 points, and evaluate how you can responsibly integrate them into your life.

Exercise

It's going to be *old news* for you to be reminded that exercising is a bit part of boosting your metabolism and burning up calories.

Unless you're born with one of those *unusually active metabolisms* which allows you to, almost freakishly, eat thousands of calories a day without weight-gain consequences, you're like the vast majority of us who need to give your metabolisms a bit of a kick through exercising.

Now, you might think that cardiovascular (aerobic) exercise is an important part of boosting your metabolism; and you'd be right!

Provided that, of course, your qualified doctor confirms that you're able to start a program of cardiovascular exercise, this is indeed the place to start. Increasing heart rate, blood circulation, body temperature, and oxygen intake/carbon dioxide exchange all send messages to the system to initiative catabolism (breaking down cells and using them for energy).

Yet if cardiovascular exercising is the place to start, does that mean that it's the place to end? *No!*

Many people, who aren't as educated as you'll be when you've finished this book, responsibly start a dedicated program of cardiovascular health, but they *don't go any further*. Not because they're lazy; but because, frankly, they don't know that there is significantly *more* that they can do in their home gym, or at the fitness club, that will boost their metabolism even more potently.

We focus upon these added activities now, below.

Build Muscle

Many people – particularly some women – are very leery about undertaking any exercise regimen that can lead to muscle building.

The old perception was that muscle building leads to *muscle bulking*, and before long, gorging forearm veins and other unwanted results. This is, frankly, not the case.

Provided that women aren't supporting their workouts with specific muscle-building supplements, there is no need to be concerned; because building lean muscle won't make them *bulk up*.

Still, however, the question remains: why would women (and, of course, men) who want to boost their metabolism focus on muscle building? Isn't cardiovascular exercising the *only* thing that matters?

Again, the answer is: No! In *addition* to a healthy and responsible cardiovascular program, muscle building is an exceptionally powerful way to boost metabolism.

How? Because a pound of muscle burns more calories than a pound of fat.

And what does this mean? It means (and get ready to stare in awe) that if you have more muscle on your body – *anywhere on your body* – you will simply burn more calories as a result.

You don't even have to *do* anything. You'll simply burn more calories, because muscle simply requires more of an energy investment.

Of course, as you can infer, if you build muscle and then leave it alone, over time, the muscle fibers will weaken and you'll lose that wonderful calorie-burning factory. But that's no problem, because all you need to do is build and maintain healthy muscle.

It may sound daunting; especially if at the moment you perceive yourself to have much more fat than muscle.

Yet the important thing for you to remember is that once you start building muscle – through any kind of strength training – your body will *itself* start burning more calories.

It has to; even while you sleep, or go to a movie, or read a book. It's like putting your calorie-burning (catabolism) program on auto-pilot.

So don't let a little (or even a lot) of extra flab, at the moment, deter you from believing that muscle building is important.

Yes, you should enjoy cardiovascular exercise too, because that's ultimately how your body is going to burn existing fat. But muscle building plays a profoundly supportive role in that pursuit.

And it's an exponential one, too: the more fat you transform into muscle, the more calories you'll burn simply to maintain that new muscle (and the wonderful cycle goes on and on!).

Interval Training

The basic weight loss *nuts and bolts* behind cardiovascular exercise (or any kind of exercise, really) is, as you know, a matter of catabolism.

Essentially, if you can engineer your body to require more energy, your body will comply by breaking cells down to deliver it; and that process (metabolism) burns calories. Simple, right?

So based on that logic, something called *interval training* neatly fits in with the overall plan. Interval training is simply a adding high-energy burning component to your exercise plan on an infrequent, or *interval*, basis.

For example, you may be at a stage where you can jog for 20 minutes every other day, and thus put your heart into a cardiovascular zone during this time.

This, obviously, is going to help you boost your metabolism and thus burn calories/energy. Yet you can actually burn *disproportionately more* calories if, during that 20 minute jog, you add a 30 second or 1 minute sprint.

Why? Because during this 30 seconds or 1 minute, you give your body a bit of a jolt.

Not an unhealthy jolt; remember, we're talking about quick bursts here, not suddenly racing around the track or through the park! By giving your body an *interval* jolt, it automatically – and somewhat unexpectedly – has to turn things up a notch.

And to compensate for your extra energy requirements, the body will burn more calories.

It's essential for you to always keep in mind that interval training *only works when it's at intervals*. This may seem like a strange thing to say (and even difficult to understand), but it's actually very straightforward.

The metabolism-boosting benefits that you enjoy as a result of interval training are primarily due to the fact that your body, suddenly, needs to find more energy.
While it was chugging along and supplying your energy needs during your cardiovascular exercising, it all of a sudden needs to go grab some more for 30 seconds or a minute; and in *that* period, it will boost your metabolism as if it were given a nice, healthy jolt.

As you can see, if you suddenly decided to extend your 30 second or 1 minute sprint into a *20 minute sprint*, you simply wouldn't experience all of the benefits.

Yes, your body would use more energy if you extend yourself to the higher range of your aerobic training zone. But your body won't necessarily get that *jolt* that only comes from interval training.

So remember: your goal with interval training is to give your body a *healthy jolt* where it suddenly says to itself:

> "Whoa! We need more energy here FAST, this person has increased their heart rate from 180 beats per minute to 190 beats per minute! Let's go to any available cell, like those fat cells down at the waist, and break them down via catabolism so that this person can get the energy that they need!"

Remember (sorry to be repetitive, but this is very important): the whole point of interval training in this way is to give your body a sudden, limited, healthy jolt where it needs more energy – quick!

If you simply increase your speed and stay there, while your body may, overall burn some more calories, it won't get that jolt.

Also bear in mind that interval training can indeed last longer than 30 seconds or a minute.

Some experts suggest that you can use interval training for 30-40 *minutes*, depending on your state of health and what your overall exercise regimen looks like.

The reason we're focusing on 30 seconds to 1 minute is simply to give you a clear understanding that interval training is a kind of mini *training within a training* program.

And, as always, *don't* overdo it with your interval training. Your goal here is to become healthier and stronger, and lose weight in that process.

You gain nothing if you run so fast or bike so hard during interval training that you hurt yourself. You will actually undermine your own health, and possibly have to stop exercising while torn muscles or other ailments heal.

Variety

They say that variety is the spice of life, and this is indeed quite true. But despite this awareness, many people don't *spice up* their exercise program; which is surprising, since doing so often leads to valuable metabolism-boosting benefits.

There are a few easy ways to add variety to your exercise program. We've already talked about interval training, and that is indeed one way to shift your body's *metabolic engine* into higher gear.

Other effective ways are to break up a longer routine into smaller parts.

For example, instead of committing to 1x1 hour workout a day, it can be metabolism-boosting to split this up into 2x30 minute workouts; or even, on some occasions, 3x20 minute workouts.

Furthermore, you can add variety into your daily exercise routine without formally *exercising*.

For example, you can take the stairs instead of the elevator. Or you can start your day with a brisk walk instead of a coffee and the newspaper.

Or, instead of parking close to the grocery store entrance, you can walk the distance between a far away parking spot and the entrance.

All of these tips provide two metabolism-boosting benefits.

Firstly, as you can easily see, they can make exercising more *fun*. While, indeed, it's important to have an exercise routine, you don't want to have a *boring* exercise routine (because then your chances of stopping are that much greater!).

So adding these new elements to your overall exercise commitment simply helps encourage you to stick with the program. And since exercising is a core part of boosting your metabolism, any technique or tip that helps you continue exercising over the long term is a wise piece of advice.

The second important benefit of variety in your exercise program leads us back to the interval training concept, discussed above.

When you add variety to your workout, your body cannot get into a *groove*. Remember: the body is a remarkable piece of work, and will always strive to do things efficiently.

Naturally, the overall state of your health (which can be influenced by genetics and other factors outside of your control) will play a role in *how* efficiently your body runs.

But regardless of how your body is put together, who what genetic influences you have to deal with, your body really likes you, and wants to do things *as efficiently as it possibly can*.

Therefore, when you start exercising, you body can start to develop a kind of expectation of energy output. It's not doing this to be lazy; it's doing this because, quite sincerely, it wants to help!

If your body starts to *predict* that you need a certain amount of energy to complete a certain task (such as jog for 20 minutes), then it will start to achieve that energy output more efficiently.

For example, when you first start jogging for, say, 2 minutes a time followed by 5 minutes of walking, your body may require a great deal of energy to help you achieve this.

And as a result, you may find yourself very out of breath or tired as your body strives to meet this increased demand. Naturally, of course, *catabolism* will be involved, and your body metabolism will increase.

But over time, say a month or so, your body will simply become more efficient. It will have become stronger, and will be able to supply your energy needs much more efficiently; you may not even break a sweat!

What's happened here is that your health has improved; your body has to *work less hard* to provide you with your energy needs.

Ironically, this can actually obscure your metabolism-boosting efforts; because, as you know, you want to tell your body to start the catabolism process. But if your body is efficiently working, it won't really dig into its reserves (e.g. fat cells) in order to provide you with the energy that you need.

So the trick is to keep *variety* in your workouts. Many people choose to cross-train for this very reason. It not only targets different muscle groups, but it keeps your body from finding a *groove* whereby it tried to help you by slowing down metabolism.

Remember: your body doesn't read books like this; it doesn't need to, and it doesn't *care*.

It has no *clue* that a speedier metabolism is *"good"* or *"bad"*. Now, as far as you and I are concerned, we know that a speedy metabolism is a *good thing* in our weight loss efforts.

But your body doesn't make this evaluation. And so it won't turn on its metabolism jets because you want it to.

You can't (unfortunately) send a memo to your body and ask it to *please speed up metabolism*.

If you *could*, then that would be amazing! But that's not reality at all. What we have to do is *force* the body to say to itself: *hey, I need to speed up metabolism because this person needs more energy!*

And one of the best ways for you to *force* the body to have this kind of thinking is to add variety to your workouts.

Lifestyle

When we come across the term *lifestyle*, we tend to think of the basic day-to-day habits that we rely on; sometimes without giving them much of a second thought. And this is indeed the case when we talk about how lifestyle influences the speed of your metabolism.

Now, quite honestly, most of us live busy lives in one form or another, and therefore it's challenging to really keep an eye on *all* of our habits.

Balancing work, family, hobbies, and other commitments often means that our lifestyle isn't so much of a *choice*, as it is a necessity.

Yet with respect to the fact that many of us face sincere limitations in our *lifestyle choices*, there are many things that we can do – little things, but important things – that can help speed up our metabolism.

So if you're a bit put-off by the term *lifestyle*, please don't skim over this section. The little things that you change in your regular, day-to-day lifestyle can indeed have the most profound influence on the speed of your metabolism, and the achievement of your short and long-term weight loss goals.

Get on the Wagon

Do you know people who carefully choose low-fat, low-calorie meal choices, are very disciplined when it comes to *not* ordering the Chef's Special pecan pie for desert, yet order a glass or two of wine with their meal?

Well, unfortunately, these people are *really* undermining their efforts to boost metabolism.

Studies show that drinking alcohol with meals actually encourages *over eating*; which means more calories that need to be burned away (or transformed into fat!).

Furthermore, many people are simply unaware that many alcoholic drinks are laden with calories; almost as much as sugary-rich soft drinks.

A bottle of beer can deliver a few hundred calories, and most cocktails are in the same range. Wine is generally considered to deliver the *least* amount of calories; but even this is a bit of a slippery slope.

Three glasses of wine can be worth 300 calories that the body simply has to *deal* with in one form or another.

The tip here isn't to stop drinking alcohol altogether (despite the title of this section). If you enjoy alcohol then there's no particular reason why you have to quit cold turkey, but you will save a bit of money and not consume as many calories.

Simply, the call here is that you become *aware* that it influences your metabolism. If you consume excess alcohol (even without becoming inebriated), you force your system to deal with more calories.

And unless you're compensating for these added calories through exercise or muscle building, catabolism cannot occur. Instead, anabolism will inevitably occur, and new cells will be created from those calories (mostly fat cells).

Zzzzzzzz.....Zzzzzzzzz

This is a toughy. Most of us don't have as much control over the amount that we sleep as we *should*. Work, family, education, housekeeping, and so many other tasks can literally prevent us from getting the amount of sleep that we need.

However, as the experts tell us, getting enough sleep actually improves metabolism. On the other hand, people who are constantly sleep deprived typically find that they have less energy to do regular, daily activities; including *digestion*.

As a result, sleep-starved people often lower their own metabolism. They simply don't have the strength to break down food efficiently, particularly carbohydrates.

This is a very difficult issue, because many people can only find time to exercise by *borrowing from* their rest time.

For example, after a long day of work and dealing with family and home commitments, a person may find that the only time they have to exercise (and thus boost their metabolism) is late at night; say around 9:00 pm, or even later. So what should one do?

Ultimately, it's a question of balance. Naturally, if you're willing to exercise, and your doctor agrees that it's healthy for you to do that, then you're *not* going to get fit by sleeping instead of exercising.

Yet with that being said, if you steal time away from your sleep/rest in order to exercise, over time, you can actually do more harm than good; because the following day, you won't have enough energy to digest what you eat. The answer to this catch-22 lies in *balance*.

You don't have to work out every night. Or perhaps you can integrate a workout into your life during the day; maybe at lunchtime or right after work.

Most fitness clubs are open very early (some are even open 24 hours), and if you choose to workout at home, you can do so in a generally affordable way (while some machines can cost thousands, basic machines that get the job done only cost a few hundred, even cheaper if they're used).

If you find that you have trouble sleeping, then this can also negatively affect the speed of your metabolism (because you won't have enough energy the following day). Insomnia and other sleep disorders are *very common problems*, and there exists a variety of support systems in place to help people get the rest that they require. Some non-medical tips to help you fall asleep include:

- o Don't eat late at night
- o Try drinking warm milk before bedtime
- o Don't turn on the TV at night
- o Try yoga or other stress-relieving practices
- o Try having a warm bath before bedtime
- o Don't exercise close to bedtime; your body can become so energized that it doesn't want to sleep!

Relax

We briefly noted *yoga* in the list of *Things to Do* above, and that brings us to another key influence of your metabolism: stress.

Believe it or not, but experts are now telling us that stress can send unwanted signals to our body; signals that lead to slower metabolism.

Essentially, what happens is that when the body is under constant stress, it releases *stress hormones* that flood the system.

These stress-related hormones actually tell the body to create larger fat cells in the abdomen. The result can be both increased weight (through increased fat cells), and a slower metabolism.

Obviously, these are *two very negative factors* in the quest to boost metabolism and lose weight. The last thing that we want is more and *bigger* fat cells in our abdomen, coupled with a diminished metabolism!

Yet this is, tragically, what happens to many people who experience constant, continuous stress. And, alas, this is *many people*; especially those of us who have to balance so many competing objectives, such as work, family, and other vital tasks.

So the advice here is indeed to "relax and chill out", and there are some simple techniques that can, and should, be added to your life.

These include walking more, listening to relaxing music, meditation, yoga, eating non-stimulating foods (e.g. no caffeine, no sugar, and so on), and building a daily regimen that includes periodic *time outs* where you can re-center yourself and de-stress.

Remember: while relaxing is good advice for anyone, it's important for you to note that stress *negatively influences metabolism.* So there is a link between how much stress you experience and your ability to break down cells and lose weight.

So if you don't want to *relax* because you don't have the time, then you should realize that your stressed-out life is probably playing a role in your weight gain/your inability to lose weight.

There's Something GOOD About This Time of the Month!?

Now here's a strange one that is *for the ladies*, only.

Studies have demonstrated that the 2-week period prior to the onset of PMS is one in which fat burning capacity is at a premium.

This is ironic indeed; because that's usually the period in which women *don't* want to workout; because their body and its emotional computer are preparing for PMS. However, studies in Australia have shown that women were able to burn off as much as 30% more fat in the 2 weeks preceding PMS.

The reason for this, researchers argue, is because this is when the female body's production of estrogen and progesterone are at their highest.

Since these hormones tell the body to use fat as a source of energy, exercising during this time can really pay off. The body will be inclined to target fat cells for catabolism.

Diet

Ah yes, diet. For most of us, our information concerning metabolism has related in one way or another to eating. Most of us have been told of metabolism-friendly foods, or metabolism *unfriendly* foods.

But really, while we may be basically aware that, all else being equal, a stalk of celery is better for your metabolism than fries with gravy, our understanding of diet and metabolism is pretty low.

To fix this, the following section looks at some powerful and scientific diet-related tips that will boost your metabolism. Indeed, as you'll soon learn, it's not merely what you eat that matters; it's when, and how, too.

Don't Hate Calories

The word calorie has a bad rap. We constantly come across *calorie reduced* or *low calorie* foods. And it's not uncommon to overhear someone gasp about the immense *calorie content* of certain foods, such as a rich and creamy desert, or a giant fast food burger.

All of this anti-calorie rhetoric therefore has made a lot of us pretty calorie-*phobic*; as soon as we see something that has lots of them, we run away. But is this wise?

Yes and no. Yes, it's wise in the sense that avoiding that double-layer chocolate fudge cake for desert is probably a good idea (actually, scratch that; it *is* a good idea).

The calories that come from the cake are really going to be the so-called *empty calorie* kind; which means that there's no real nutritional value that your body can squeeze out and make use of.

But in the bigger picture, it's *unwise* for your metabolism to become calorie-avoidant.

Why? Because your body is a marvelous machine that tries, at all times, to do what it can to make your life easier.

Indeed, while it may not always function at optimal levels (for a variety of reasons, including genetics), it still tries to do its very best. The body, for all of its limitations and so forth, is *not* a lazy thing!

With this in mind, the body is always trying to keep is alive and functioning in the manner that it deems to be healthiest.

And that's why if you suddenly decrease the amount of calories that you need, your body won't try to *do more with less*. In other words, your body won't respond in the way that you want it to: it won't necessarily provoke catabolism and thus reduce weight and fat cells.

Instead, your smart and wise body will try to *keep you alive* by slowing down its metabolism. It will simply believe that something is wrong – maybe you're trapped somewhere without food – and it will just begin to become very stingy with energy.

So what's the end result? If your body needs 2000 calories a day to survive, and you suddenly give it only 1000, it *won't* begin to burn off 1000 calories worth of cells that you have lying around on your love handles.

Instead, your body will *slow down its metabolism*. It will really try and get as much energy out of those 1000 calories, because it doesn't want to waste anything.

Physically, you'll naturally feel more tired because your body is being very miserly with energy, and will devote its 1000-calorie ration to essential systems, like blood and oxygen supply (and others).

Metabolically, you won't be burning off extra calories. In fact, you can actually *gain weight* by dramatically reducing your calorie intake!

The flipside of this, of course, is that you should consume a daily caloric intake that is proportionate to your body size, type, and weight loss goals.

And then, once you determine the amount of calories that you need (probably with the aid of a qualified nutritionist or fitness expert); you can provide that to your body via healthy, efficient calories.

For example, if your body needs 1500 calories per day, and one slice of double-fudge chocolate cake delivers a whopping 500 of those, then you can see that eating just one of these slices will take up a full 1/3rd of your daily caloric needs; and that's not good!

On the other hand, you can see that drinking a tasty fruit smoothy made with yogurt and nuts can deliver half as many calories, but provide you with essential nutrients, vitamins, and other elements that your body needs to healthily do its work.

Eat More?

Fresh on the heels of the discussion on calories, it's also helpful to note that eating frequently throughout the day can be very good for boosting metabolism. There are a couple of reasons for this.

The first reason is that people who tend to eat throughout the day do considerably less *snacking*. As a result, they tend to avoid the potato chips or candy bars that they might otherwise consume if they suddenly felt *hungry*.

People who eat throughout the day don't tend to experience severe *hunger pangs*, because they don't reach that stage.

The second reason, and the one that you can probably guess based on your understanding of metabolism, is that by eating throughout the day, you are constantly keeping your metabolism in motion.

It's kind of like having a generator run all the time; it will simply use more electricity than if you powered it on 3 times a day.

Now, it goes without saying (but we should say it anyway just in case!) that just because it's *good* for metabolism-boosting to eat frequently, this *doesn't* mean that you can eat *junk* all day long!

Rather, if you choose to eat more frequently, then you'll certainly need to be very aware of *what* you eat; because you can easily exceed your required amount of daily calories if you don't keep an eye on this.

That's why, if your plan is to follow the eat-more-to-burn-more approach, then you should keep a food journal that notes what you eat (and drink of course) throughout the day.

You should not merely know the calorie levels of what you eat, but you should know the overall nutritional values, too.

For example, if you're on target to eat 50 grams of protein per day, then you want to make sure you reach this target and not exceed it (or come in below it).

In other words, merely focusing on calories is only half of the job. You will need to ensure that you're eating enough protein, carbohydrates, fats (the good unsaturated kind!), and the other vitamins and minerals that your body needs in order to function at optimal levels.

Eat Early

We've all heard that *breakfast is the most important meal of the day*. And in terms of boosting your metabolism, this is indeed the case! There are a couple of reasons why eating a hearty and healthy breakfast can boost metabolism and lead to weight loss goals.

The first reason is that people who eat breakfast are much less inclined to snack throughout the morning. For example, if you had a good breakfast of fruit and low-sugar cereal in the morning, your chances of visiting the vending machine at work around 10:30am diminish significantly.

Of course, as you recall from our previous discussion on eating more frequently, this doesn't mean that you shouldn't eat something between breakfast and lunch.

It simply means that, since you won't be extremely hungry at 10:30am (because you skipped breakfast), you'll be less inclined to eat *anything* that you get your hands on; such as a nice donut that your co-worker was kind enough to offer you.

In other words, by starting your day in a nutritious way, you'll have more control over *what* you eat throughout the day.

The second reason is more aligned with metabolism-boosting. Studies have shown that metabolism slows during sleep, and doesn't typically get going again until you eat.

Therefore, starting the day with breakfast is like kickstarting your metabolism. You'll actually burn more calories throughout the day, simply by eating breakfast (hey, who knew?!).

Remember: as you eat your breakfast, control both the portion and the contents. You don't want to eat to the point of complete fullness; because, remember, you want to eat throughout the day and you won't be able to do that if you're *stuffed*.

At the same time, beware of high-fat breakfasts. Studies have shown that high-fat breakfasts, such as those that include bacon and sausage, not only deliver *lots of calories* (there are 9 calories for every gram of fat, as compared to 4 for every gram of carbohydrates and proteins, respectively).

But they also can make you very hungry again, very soon! So in addition to having ingested a lot of fat (and hence a lot of calories), you'll typically find yourself rather ravenous again in a few hours.

Alternatively, breakfasts that are high in fiber take longer to digest, and thus, the body won't be hungry again for a while.

This is something to bear in mind; and it may explain why many people who eat breakfast find themselves *painfully hungry* by lunchtime; it's not their "overactive metabolism" at work; it's the high fat content, which has been swiftly digested.

Befriend Protein and Good Carbs

There is a *dizzying* array of things that you can eat these days. Truly, a trip to the grocery store can be an adventure. Everywhere you turn, there's yet another food promising you *healthy this* or *weight loss that*.

Added to this confusion is that there are some foods that are beneficial for metabolic boosting, and some that *aren't*; and the differences aren't always well-known. Fortunately, we're going to tackle this problem right now and describe the three basic food groups/types that are indeed good for a speedy metabolism.

In terms of protein, studies have shown that having enough protein in your system can actually increase the speed of your metabolism. This is because protein is difficult to break down. Or rather, it *requires more energy* to break down. It's like feeding the body a knot; it needs a bit of time to unravel it.

And, as you know, when your body spends time on something, it *spends energy* (calories). And so the more time it can spend breaking down protein, the more calories that it uses.

Different people will require different amounts of protein on a daily basis. Those who exercise and build muscle will typically need more than the average amount, too.

The USFDA Food Guide suggests around 50 grams of protein a day for a *reasonably active adult*.

Keep in mind (not that you don't already have *enough* to remember, but...) that there are different sources of protein: some lean, and some high in fat. Fast food burgers may deliver up to 20 grams of protein (sometimes more), but they also deliver a great deal of *fat*; which makes them almost nutritionally worthless.

The benefits you enjoy from the protein are far outweighed by the immense fat intake; which, for some fast food burgers, can exceed 40 grams! And that's *not* including the fries (we won't even go there!).

So the thing to do is ensure that your source of protein derives from *lean* protein. Typically, protein from *some* fish and chicken is lean; though not all of it.

If you're a vegetarian, or simply looking for non-meat lean protein alternatives, low-fat cheese, legumes (lentils), and yogurt are all good sources. Simply check the food labels to determine if the source of protein is lean (doesn't deliver high fat content), or fatty.

In terms of carbohydrates, there probably isn't a more battered around micronutrient than this. It's gone from being the greatest thing in weight loss history, to one of the most reviled.
And really, it's not the fault of the innocent carbohydrate! It's really just a matter of information and knowledge, instead of speculation.

The thing to remember is that when carbohydrates are refined, such as white bread and potatoes, they are what the diabetic world refers to as *high glycemic index (GI) foods*, because they require spikes in insulin in order to be digested.

As you may know, when insulin is released into the system, it promotes the storage of fat; and some experts believe that it also pushes down metabolic speed (which makes sense).

Therefore, the *good* kinds of carbohydrate to consume are those that are high in fiber, and those from fruit and vegetable sources.

Why? Because these sources of carbohydrates don't score high on the glycemic index. In other words, they don't cause a spike in insulin levels, and therefore, they don't promote fat storage.

Conclusion

We've come a long way! We now actually know more about the metabolism, and how to increase metabolic speed, than most people; and we're therefore in a position to put that information to *good use*.

We've learned that the metabolism is a process and not an actual body part.

It harmonizes two essential bodily functions: converting food into cells/tissues, and breaking cells down to provide energy. We learned that the former process is known as *anabolism*, and the latter is *catabolism*.

Indeed, it's this latter process that influences our ability to lose weight, and to keep it from coming back!

Yet going beyond the biological basics, we also learned of 3 integrated aspects of speeding up metabolism and losing weight.

These aspects were categorized in terms of: *exercise, lifestyle, and diet*. And within each of these 3 categories were a total of 11 important, practical, and quite easy ways to boost metabolism.

Now, indeed, it's the time for *action*; for as they say, wisdom is the result of experience, not study! Obviously, of course, it was essential for us to understand this subject and how it relates to boosting metabolism. So in that light, study is invaluable. But now you're equipped with the knowledge that you need.

The next step – boosting your metabolism – is all up to you.   Good luck, have fun, and enjoy your better, *leaner* healthier life!

A Final Word: Common Metabolism-Boosting Myths

The SparkDiet resource center[ii] has consulted fitness experts to find the 4 most prevalent myths concerning metabolism and metabolism-boosting.

Since this book has been about reality and *not* myths, we didn't cover any of them in the actual book. Yet, considering how common these myths are, it can indeed be useful for you to know them; and to *know* that they're myths.

That way, if you come across them in a magazine, at a fitness club, or just from the well-intentioned but misguided advice of a friend, you can confidently say (or at least just *think*): sorry, but that's a myth; I'm not going to fall for that one!

Myth #1: Diet Pills

The general consensus on diet pills are contained in two powerful words: BUYER BEWARE.

The problem here is that many makers of diet pills offer claims that simply aren't realistic; and if you read the fine-print of most of these advertisements, you'll see that they're really too good to be true. Little notes like *the claims made in this advertisement are not typical* should be enough of a wake-up call to realize that there's more to the story.

In some cases, diet pills can help *boost* metabolism temporarily. This, however, can be risky and generally shouldn't be done without a doctor's say-so. Unfortunately, people can become somewhat addicted to diet pills, and this can lead to disaster.

And before we go onto myth #2, remember that some diet pills are *water loss pills*. That is, they are diuretics that promote water loss, usually through excess urination. The jury on water-loss diet pills is somewhat less open-minded than diet pills in general: THEY DON'T WORK!

Seriously: water loss diet pills are built on the premise that you'll lose weight through water. And, yes, that's true: if you urinate 15 times a day, you're physically going to weigh less.

But this is *not* actual weight loss! This is merely unhealthy temporary weight loss, and it will come roaring back the minute that water stores are replenished through diet.

Or, even harder to comprehend, if a person taking these water pills fails to restore their body's fluid needs, they can actually suffer dehydration; which can, and has, led to coma and death.

Myth #2: Drop Caloric Intake

As we discussed earlier in this book (but it's so important that it deserves an encore here at the end), trying to lose weight by drastically cutting down calories *doesn't work*; in fact, it's unhealthy.

The thing to remember is that the body's ability to lose weight is not controlled by calories. Calories are the input. The real control mechanism is that famous concept that you've become very familiar with: *metabolism.*

Calories are merely units of energy. It's how your body *deals* with that energy that determines whether weight is gained or lost.

So with that being said, cutting down your caloric intake to, say, 1000 calories a day isn't necessarily going to help you lose weight; because *it doesn't necessarily change your metabolism.*

Indeed, as you know, if you slow down your caloric intake, your body – which is always trying to help you in the best way that it knows how – *will slow down its metabolism.*

Really, it makes sense: the body says that something has gone wrong; instead of the 2000 calories that it needs, it's only getting 1000. The body doesn't know *why* this is happening; it doesn't know that you want to lose weight.

It just senses that something is wrong; perhaps you're trapped in a cave or something, or stuck in a snowstorm. So the body, trying to help you, will slow down its metabolism; it will do its best to slow down the conversion rate, so that you have as much energy *on hand* as possible.

Now, if your body was able to read this book and you could say: look, please just do what you normally do, but do it with 1000 fewer calories a day for a while, then we might actually get somewhere.

But the body doesn't work that way. It *won't* help you lose weight if you dramatically cut down on calories.

It will slow down metabolism, and (here's the worst part), if and when you ever increase calories again, your body will have to deal with that *via a slower metabolic engine.* So you can actually *gain weight* if, after cutting down your calories for a period of time, you find that you consume extra calories (say while on vacation or something).

Myth #3: Low Intensity Workouts

It's fair to say that *any* exercise is better than *no* exercise. So if you lead a sedentary lifestyle, then even walking around your block for 10 minutes a day is going to something positive for your body and its metabolism.

True, that difference may be imperceptible to the naked eye (or it may not?), the bottom line is that exercise is good.

Yet with this being said, some people believe that they should perform low-intensity workouts *even when* they could be performing more high-intensity workouts.

That is, instead of jogging for 20 minutes with their heart at the top end of their aerobic zone, they opt for low-intensity jogs that barely break a sweat.

Low intensity workouts simply don't lead to a faster metabolism; they *can't*. Remember, as we discussed very early in this book, metabolism is a *process*.

And that process is really one of two types: taking energy and making cells (*anabolism*), or breaking cells down to make energy (*catabolism*).

If you don't achieve a high-intensity workout, your body can't tap achieve catabolism; it won't need to. And the only way your body is going to go and break down existing cells is if it *needs to*.

So keep this in mind as you exercise, either at home or at a gym. Low intensity workouts are better than *nothing at all*; and they may be necessary if you're recovering from injury, or just starting out on the exercise journey.

But once you reach a level of basic fitness, only high intensity (aerobic) workouts will make a difference in terms of your metabolism. High intensity workouts force your body to find energy to help you maintain that level of exercise; and it does so through catabolism.

Speeding up your metabolism and achieving your weight loss goals involved a certain degree of focus; after all, there's a lot of things competing for your attention (including that delicious Chef's Special pecan pie!), and you certainly need to be able to keep your eye on the goal in order to maintain your program.

Yet sometimes too much focus can be a bad thing; and some dieters understand this all too well.

Remember: speeding up your metabolism is a *holistic* effort that includes exercise, lifestyle, and diet changes.

Focusing on only one of these at the expense of the others (either one or both) can be detrimental. In fact, in some cases, it can be counter-productive.

So the myth here is that you *shouldn't* go all out and focus on becoming an exercise guru, and then move onto lifestyle, and then to diet.

You have to integrate *all 3* aspects into your life *at the same time*. True, based on your unique situation, you will likely emphasize one more than the others. That's fine and normal. But it's a myth – and a mistake – to ignore any one of these.

It takes all three to speed up your metabolism, and to get you to your weight loss goals for the long-term.

[i] Lavine, Hallie. "14 Ways to Boost your Metabolism".
iVillage.com.http://magazines.ivillage.com/redbook/dh/diet/articles/0,,284479_577038,00.html

[ii] SparkDiet. http://sparkpeople.com/resource/nutrition_articles.asp?id=476